Simple and Fit

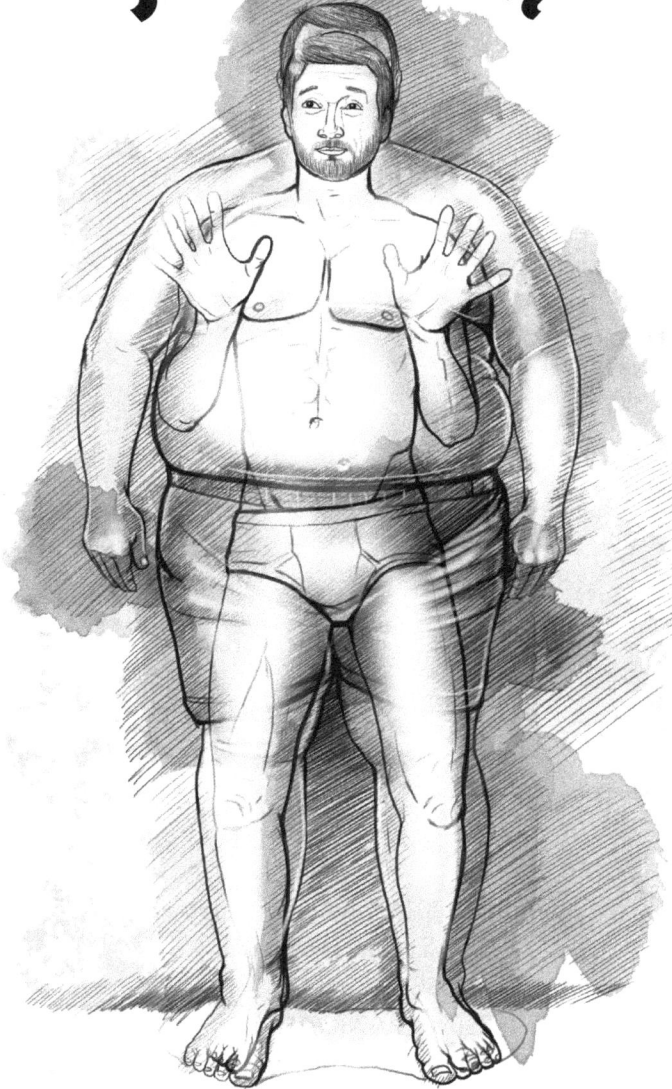

BY JONATHAN PAUL ANKIEWICZ

CONTENTS

ACKNOWLEDGMENTS

I just wanted to take a second and thank my parents.
Thank you, Mom and Dad, for showing me that anything can
be accomplished. And that everything is simple, as long as you
break it down to the basics and apply discipline.
There isn't anything you can't do in this world without effort.

FOREWORD

If the premise of this book intrigued you—a simplified look at what it takes to get fit—welcome to the club, because you are likely like many of us who have often been overwhelmed by the avalanche of information and misinformation available on this topic. Everywhere you turn, it seems, there is an absolute mountain of new research or advice about "how to live a healthy lifestyle" and "have a body just like (this or that celebrity) you see on TV."

Putting aside celebrities, who have the cash on hand for their own army of personal trainers and dieticians, you have probably noticed some athletic, fit people around you in the course of your own day. These are the real people—whether they are friends, cow-orkers, acquaintances, or just someone you run into—who make you think to yourself, "Wow, I'd love to have a body like that!"

If so, I have some great news for you. Those muscular, fit people who look like they can grace the cover of a magazine? There's no dif-ference between them and you. Really.

Sure, some among us have incredible genetic gifts and were seemingly born with six-pack abs, but more often than not, someone with a great physique has simply put forth the effort to improve his or her eating habits and exercise regularly.

Okay, so there is one difference: They were introduced to the tenets of a healthier lifestyle at some point. They've learned some key rules to live by, and they just tapped the willpower that, believe it or not, is ingrained in all of us and needs to be developed and nurtured.

You may stop at this point and say, "Jonathan, you're totally understating the role of genetics in this. Some people I know can eat anything they want, and they always look incredible."

Yes, genetics, as I said, gives some lucky souls a leg up. But it's a small edge. It may give them a faster metabolism, so they burn fat faster than average. Or they can gain appreciable muscle with less effort. But what you may not realize is that even those with solid genetic traits have their own hurdles to overcome. For one thing, such ease of staying in shape can tend to make them a bit lazier and thus more likely to lose it quickly as the inevitable metabolic slowdowns of aging occur. They may also plateau faster, while someone with lesser genetics—but who is bound and determined to improve—will pass them up. Sure, it may be "a nice problem to have," but all of us have our own challenges to face.

In any case, your focus here should be solely on yourself, because it doesn't matter what obstacles others face, or what advantages they have. It only matters what you're dealing with and thus what you need to do to create the dream body you want.

That's where I hope this short, simple book comes in. I wanted to give you a clear, concise overview of the basic rules anyone can follow to live a healthy, fit life. And I want to do it in a way that's not overwhelming, as can happen when you try to research this topic for yourself. The amount of information you sometimes come across can be so detailed and steeped in scientific jargon that it seems they are writing in a different language. Some of these sources make it sound as if you have to study the art of fitness for years and years before you actually start to learn the ropes and apply it seamlessly to your everyday life. It can be downright discouraging, I know.

I'm here to tell you, however, it doesn't need to be complicated. Not at all. Depending on your current situation, it may be hard to believe that a few rules can change your life, but I know it can. I've seen it happen firsthand. I chose to write this book because I love seeing people live a healthy lifestyle, and because I want the so-called "secret" of fitness to be out: that being fit and looking like a superhero is indeed *simple*.

YOUR BODY IS A MACHINE —
IT NEEDS TO BE WELL MAINTAINED.

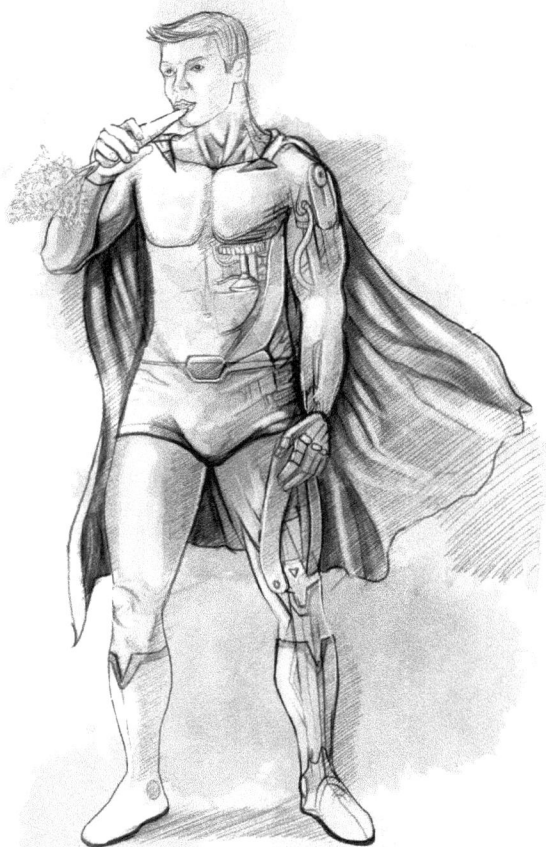

The first thing you need to change before changing anything else is your mind-set. You need to approach the idea of your body in a different way. You need to be aware of it and not take it for granted anymore.

I've found that it helps to start thinking of your body as a machine. How? Well, it requires fuel like a machine. It also does exactly what you tell it to do, like a machine. It has standard functions, like a machine. For example, if you feed it enough, it grows, and if you feed it too much, it gets too large.

One important difference? The human body doesn't come with an operator's manual. Creating that is your responsibility. So that is the mission as you push forward on this quest to improve your health and physical attributes—along the way, you want to pay attention to how your body responds and reacts and learn from that, so you know what works for you and what doesn't. You're going to want to begin carrying a journal with you wherever you go.

DOING ONE EXERCISE TO OBLIVION IS NEVER THE ANSWER.

If you watch enough infomercials, you'd think that crafting a set of incredible abs could be accomplished by rep after rep of an exercise.

Truth is, you could do two million crunches and not get a set of washboard abs. I'm not saying this to discourage you; I'm telling you because the key is to work smarter—not harder then you have to.

In the case of abs, or any part of your body you want to improve, doing tons of reps and lots of workouts will make you stronger, but if you also want definition, you need to view the whole picture of fitness, and that means recuperation and nutrition, too.

Thus, to see the fruits of your hard work, you need to reduce your body fat via exercise, clean eating, and rest.

Just keep in mind that a holistic approach is the only one that works. You can't just do one part, ignore the others, and expect to make the progress you want. Think of it this way:

- **Food** is the building supplies and energy source your body needs.
- **Exercise** creates the need for muscle building/repair and fat burning.
- **Sleep** is when your body uses the supplies to rebuild and burn. A time where it does all of the processing.

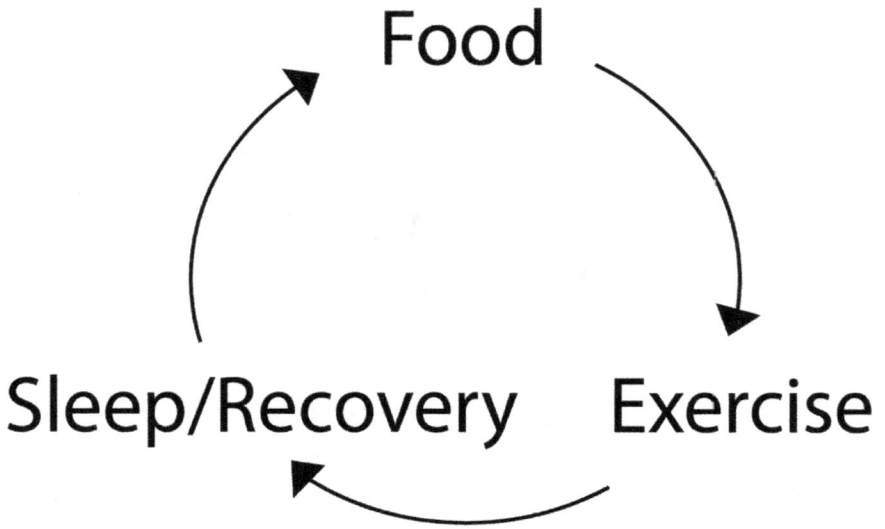

WATER IS LIFE— 60 PERCENT OF IT, ACTUALLY.

You've probably heard the advice to hydrate since way back in your school days, but its importance goes beyond making sure you don't pass out in gym class.

Water, in fact, is the number-one key factor in the proper functioning of your body. It's critical in the all functions of humans, from the simplest to the most complex. It is used in the chemical construction and deconstruction of muscle, fat, bone, organs, and more. It's also used to regulate temperature. The human body, all told, is made up of roughly 60 percent water.

So, you may think, I just make sure I take in enough liquids, and I'm set. But just because a drink is in "liquid" form doesn't mean it will actually serve to hydrate you. Some drinks act like a diuretic—in other words, they will cause your body to lose water by excreting it, meaning drinking too much can lead to dehydration! For example, caffeinated beverages like coffee and soda can be counterproductive in this way.

This doesn't mean you can't enjoy a cup of your favorite caffeinated beverage. It just means you need to be sure to take in some pure water along with it. A good general rule that I've found is to be sure to have two eight-ounce glasses of water for every one of coffee, tea, or soda you may drink.

Think of your water hydration level as a meter for your
body's performance. When
your hydration meter begins
to drop, your body's natural performance begins to
drop as well. When you get to
three-fourths of your optimal
hydration level, your body
is going to perform
at 75 percent of your
body's abilities. It can
be hard to notice
if you're not pay-
ing close attention
during strenuous activity,
but if you pay attention to the
signals, you'll feel it in your muscles and joints.

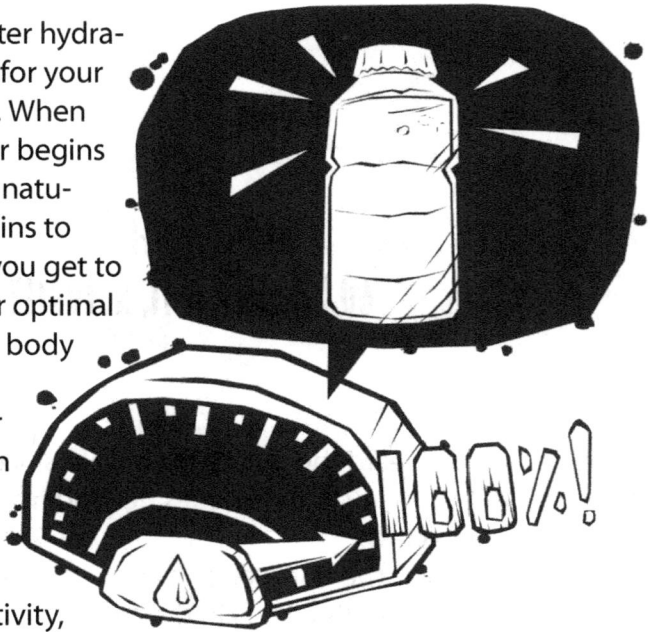

Unfortunately, we don't have a mechanism to tell us we're going
to be thirsty soon. Feeling thirsty is a signal from your body that you
need to hydrate, but there's a catch. Thirst is a late signal, and you're
already a little late, because at that point you're already at some point
of dehydration. To avoid that, keep water on hand, and sip it all day
long.

Exactly how much water per day is enough is the subject of constant debate. Standard nutritional guidelines say eight eight-ounce
glasses of water per day.

But think about what happens when you exercise a lot. You
sweat, right? And during that time, you want your body to perform
at its peak. So I suggest going a little further than simply accepting
sixty-four ounces at face value. Do a little calculation: divide your
weight in half, and drink that resulting figure times one ounce of

water per day. So if you're a two-hundred-pound male, aim for a hundred ounces. Or to look at it another way, drink one ounce of water for every two pounds you weigh.

If you haven't been drinking that much water regularly, the reality is, you'll be visiting the restroom many times as your body adjusts, so be ready. But while you're there, you can also easily gauge whether your water intake is doing as intended: if your pee is very yellow and has an odor to it, you're dehydrated. If it's clearer and odor-free, you're taking in enough.

Of course, you don't want to carry a measuring cup wherever you go. So here's a quick breakdown of typical serving sizes as they relate to ounces:

Water serving sizes:
Coffee cup—8 ounces
Tall kitchen glass—12 ounces
One-liter bottle—33.8 ounces
One quart—32 ounces
One gallon—128 ounces

A final note: If you choose to hydrate with a sports drink, you should dilute it, because the sugar content in these drinks is usually very high. So add one equal part of water to each serving.

DON'T LOSE SIGHT OF WHAT'S REALLY IMPORTANT TO MAKE PROGRESS.

It has been said that as much of 80 percent of body-building success isn't training, as one might first guess. As an old body-building saying goes, "Your body is built in the kitchen." You can work out as hard and as smart as you can, but without the nutritional building blocks on hand for your body to react and respond to, those actions in the gym will just go for naught.

However, that doesn't mean you necessarily need to become a nutritional scientist to achieve your aims. I'd get some argument from plenty of my peers, but based on everything I've learned through research and experience, I can say without a doubt that it's not so much what you eat as how you eat.

In other words, it truly boils down to calories into the body versus calories out, or activity levels. While I wouldn't recommend it because of the health ramifications, when it comes to fat loss, you can eat foods that are lousy for you, but as long as you take in less than your daily caloric requirements—what your body burns daily—you won't get fat.

Of course, there is a catch: "whatever you want to eat" doesn't mean "all you can eat." One large fast-food hamburger with a large fries and a regular Coke meets the entire daily caloric intake for an average 150-pound person. That means, if you choose that meal, that's all you can eat for the entire day, from the time you wake up until the time you hit the pillow at night.

I don't like to see people getting caught up in counting calories. It's complicated and time consuming, and unless you're under 12 percent body fat already, and you're trying to dial in the last few percentage ticks downward, you shouldn't have to. Instead, just do your best to steer clear of highly processed foods, fast foods, and binge eating. If you keep your diet pretty clean (i.e., free of high-fat and high-sugar foods), stick to smaller portions, plan out small meals spaced two to three hours apart throughout the day, and don't eat a big meal near bedtime, you should be fine and make progress.

As you do this, it will also help you to learn more about nutrition. After all, the more you know, the better choices you can make. So I'm sharing the following information as a basic guide, so you can be more aware in making your dietary choices.

STOKE YOUR METABOLIC FURNACE TO BURN MORE CALORIES THAN YOU TAKE IN.

As I stated, nutrition for weight loss is all about calories in versus calories out. "Calories in" refers to the food you eat, and "calories out" is the energy you burn during exercise or your daily routine.

This "burning" process is essentially your metabolism—a chemical process within your body that's essential for the maintenance of life. In extremely simple terms, metabolism is the process by which some substances (i.e., food) are broken down to create energy to fuel vital processes and muscle activity.

More simply put, your body takes the food you eat and uses it to provide you energy throughout the day. It also uses it to build and rebuild muscle.

This calorie burning is a constant process, occurring day and night with no rest. A measure of this is referred to as the "basal metabolic rate." Also understand that your body is rarely if ever in complete homeostasis (a point of perfect balance). You're either burning more calories than you're taking in, or you're burning less, and the excess is being put toward muscle repair or stored as fat.

So the goal is to make sure your metabolism is humming along optimally. Some may look at this so far and think, "Okay, calories in versus calories out. So I can just starve myself and lose weight, right?"

But no, it is not that easy. That's because the human body has mechanisms in place to help save itself from starvation. After all, the goal throughout the evolutionary process has been survival, not six-pack abs, so your body processes are geared to keep the body strong and stable for as long as possible, even in times of low food intake.

Thus, when you starve yourself, your body won't conveniently tap your body fat. No, instead it'll seek out the easiest calories to burn it can, and that means muscle tissue.

This will keep you alive if you're a hunter and don't know where your next meal is coming from, but these days, that ancient human physiology doesn't help very much for those who are after a cut, muscular physique.

Muscle is key, and losing it will derail your progress. That's because muscle is not only aesthetically pleasing, but it serves as a metabolic furnace. Muscle tissue burns calories, even at rest. The more muscle you have, the more high-powered your metabolic rate is. But if you lose your muscle mass to starvation diets, your body becomes less and less efficient, and you end up with exactly what you don't want: a body made up of metabolically inactive fat.

UNDERSTAND WHAT YOUR BODY CAN USE TO CREATE ENERGY.

Calories are the measurement used to define energy. Your body can receive this unit of energy from the food you eat, or by breaking down its existing muscle and fat stores, which makes sense, since it is calories you took in previously that built those structures in the first place.

For the sake of what you're trying to achieve as far as your physique is concerned, you want to avoid that muscle-tissue breakdown at all costs. When your body is in that mode, it's called "catabolism," while muscle building is considered an "anabolic" state. You'd prefer that your body just break down the fat stores instead for energy.

In supersimple terms, the idea behind eating and exercising is to put your body in the right state: one in which you take in enough calories so that you don't enter starvation mode, and you have the protein and energy on hand to repair muscle. In addition, you want to set the stage so that your body naturally taps your fat for its extra energy needs.

It sounds like you're juggling a lot, I know. But while the human body is a complex machine, what you have to do to set the stage for muscle gain and fat loss is not. It comes back to the "calories in, calories out" mantra: Eat a little less than your body burns in a normal day, exercise with weights to spur positive changes in your muscle mass, and do some form of cardiovascular activity daily for your health.

In other words, the goal for prime weight loss is to create just enough of a calorie shortage that your body only consumes fat but not so much that it takes muscle, too.

It is a delicate balance, admittedly, because if you starve yourself instead of taking a more moderate approach, everything you're trying to do will go for naught. The body is designed to sense starvation and combat it by storing everything it can as fat. That way, the reasoning goes, if starvation happens again, it'll be even more prepared with those fat stores to tap. Calories will be shunted away from the regular role of muscle repair. Starvation diets actually lead to fat and weight gain in the long run. That's why they always fail.

KICK-START
YOUR METABOLISM.

Your metabolism is fueled by calories and runs hotter or cooler based on numerous factors that are a little different for everyone. It's based on genetics, weight, muscle mass, and your daily eating habits.

Can I tell you exactly how many calories your metabolism burns? Admittedly, no. You'll have to use trial and error to figure it out so that you can write the operator's manual for your own body. But for now, as you are just getting into fitness and health, there is no need to pay attention to specific calories.

When you eat a meal, your body takes all of those calories and uses them to run all of your functions. Storing energy, making energy, and using energy. Muscle building and repair. It also dips in to your stored fat to meet all of the body's needs, assuming you're eating in that sweet spot of enough food, but just shy.

Every meal you eat begins its process of digestion as you take your first bite. Think of your stomach as a fuel tank. You need to empty it before you can fill it again. Because everyone's bodies are different, the processing times vary, due to the quality of food we consume and our genetic abilities. Healthier clean foods tend to digest faster and easier then highly processed foods.

Here is where the food monitoring gets tricky. You're going to need your operator's manual journal for this. If you refuel your tank too early, your body will take those extra calories and try to store them as fat. If you take too long to refuel your tank, then your body will begin to worry and start initiating starvation mode tactics and begin to store the calories as fat. It is your job to begin listening to your body and determine the best range for it.

Now don't get worried or caught up in the idea of calories and how much to eat and the exact minute to eat. Your body will tell you everything you need to know. Just listen to it, but make sure you give it some time to process. It should take twenty to forty-five minutes before your body has the ability to signal you that you ate to much or too little. Please note: as you listen, it is your job to determine the difference between a hunger and a craving. Cravings are for a particular food. Hunger is when you feel the urge to eat. You need to fight the cravings and obey the hunger.

To learn your own body's rhythms, you can experiment by setting up mealtimes spaced anywhere from two to four hours apart. Then see how your physique and energy levels respond. This is where a food journal comes in very handy, and it is highly recommended.

Athletes often eat five to seven small meals per day, spaced two to three hours apart. Based on such a window, and thinking you're awake for about fifteen hours a day on average, that's the number of meals that "fit" into such a window. That's a pro, though—you may find two to three hours apart is too close, and you're taking in too many calories overall, even with smaller meals. Again, experiment and watch the signs of progress in the mirror and on the scale.

There are reams of scientific data behind all of this—but this is why you picked up this book, I imagine, so you don't need to read mountains of studies to figure out what to do!

With your number of meals in mind, you'll also want to figure out how much to eat per meal. Unfortunately, I cannot provide specific advice on this front. As everyone is different, anything I give as far as hard and fast rules can't possibly work for everyone. Instead of setting concrete guidelines that may help only 10 percent of the readers, I'd rather steer you toward designing your own, thus helping everyone.

So here's what to do. Start a daily journal and write down

- what you ate at every meal;
- what time you ate;
- how you felt after you ate (twenty to forty-five minutes later);
- how you felt at the end of the day;
- how you felt first thing in the morning;
- your weight—daily, in the a.m., before the first meal;
- any other factors about how your body looks and your progress toward your personal goals.

You'll want to continually monitor this data and make changes as warranted. You're looking to see if you feel like you have more energy. Do you just feel cleaner and healthier, or do you feel sluggish, slow-witted, still hungry, or even stuffed after eating?

After a couple of weeks, you can start looking for trends in your weight—is it going up, dropping, or stationary? As you keep track of all of this data, you will learn how your body reacts to specific foods and eating methods, and you can make adjustments to your diet based on your findings.

CONTROL YOUR PORTIONS.

As I said, I'm not going to give you a specific diet plan, because one diet plan isn't going to work for everyone. Those who design a diet and say, "It worked for me," or "it worked for such-and-such celebrity," isn't giving a true picture of success. They don't mention the 90 percent of users for whom the diet did nothing.

Diets need to be tailored for your specific lifestyle and your body's ability to process foods. This is why personal trainers can be so successful at their jobs, as opposed to the results a typical person gets out of a fitness DVD. It's because a trainer has the ability to individualize the diets and closely monitor progress as his or her client works through the process.

What I can help you determine is portion control. This isn't the same as calorie counting. If you're interested in weighing your foods and counting every calorie you eat, go ahead and try those methods. But keep in mind, those require a lot of tracking and math. If you're unfamiliar with the methods of calorie counting, I recommend you seek a professional trainer to help get you on track.

For me, portion control can do a lot of that work, and more easily. Portion control alone will make a positive impact on an enormous number of you reading this. You will see drastic changes in your body. A warning: you may experience plenty of hunger at first, especially if you are used to eating a lot, but if that's the case, I implore you to stay the course. After a while, you will become accustomed to eating proper-size meals, and at that point you can go back to trusting your body's signals telling you when you're hungry and when you're full.

When choosing your meals, I recommend starting with the recommended food groups from the USDA, picking—at most—only one serving per group. If you find yourself needing a second helping, try to stick mainly with the protein and vegetables.

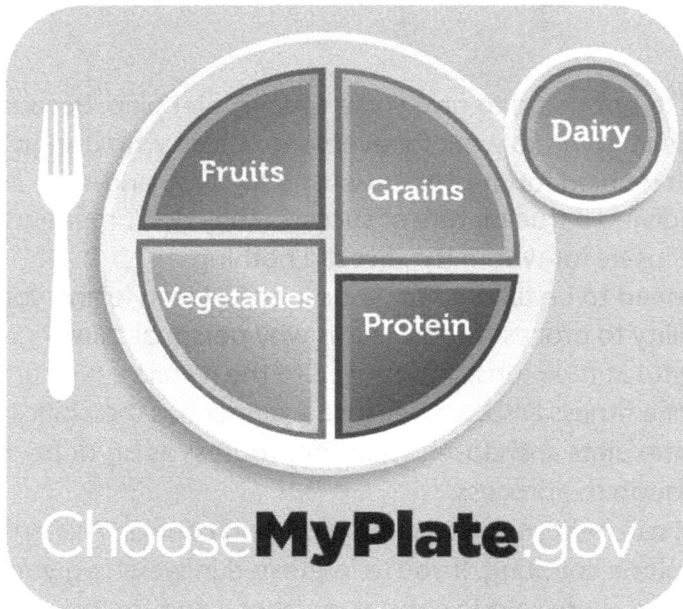

Familiarize yourself with what these portions look like in real life. Once you can accurately gauge these portions by sight, when a meal is placed in front of you, it won't be hard to determine what to eat and what to take home in a doggy bag. How to determine the proper portion of food?

The average serving size of any given meat is roughly three to four ounces. Visually this is about the same size as a computer mouse or a cell phone.

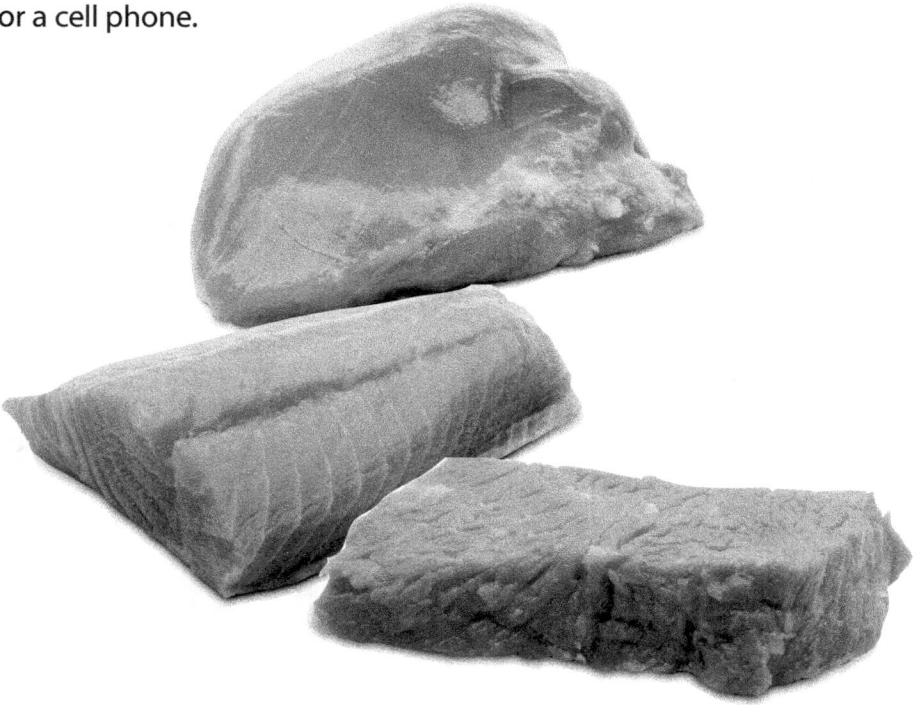

The average serving size of vegetables tends to range from about half of a cup to a full eight-ounce cup of diced-up veggies. But if you're ever still feeling hungry after a meal, feel free to eat almost any green vegetable as much as you want, as they tend to be low in calories. Lettuce, broccoli, cauliflower, spinach, and asparagus are just a few examples.

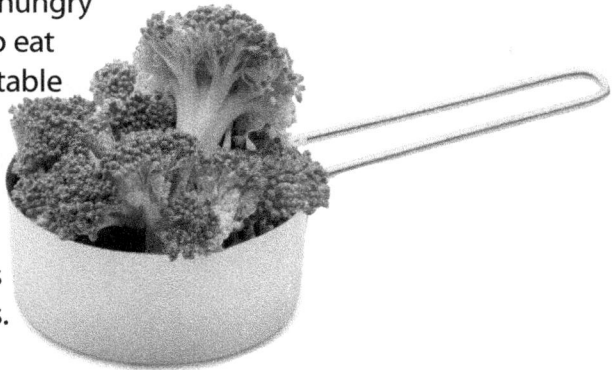

Note that it does not include salad dressing or dipping sauces, which are often loaded with calories.

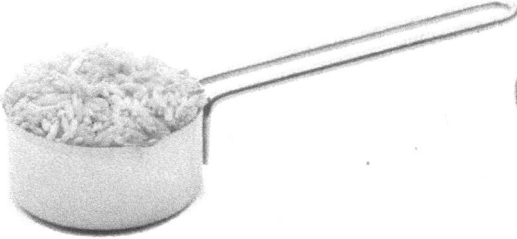

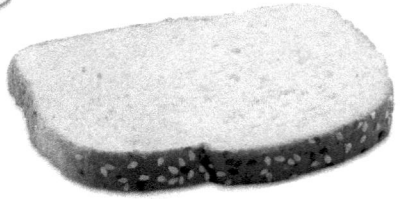

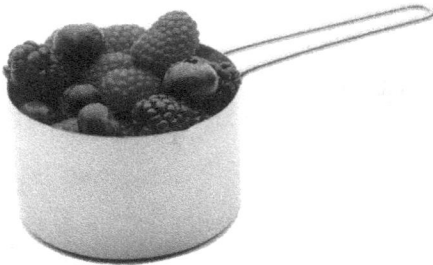

An average serving of grains is roughly one slice of bread to a half cup, while the average serving size of fruit is about four ounces.

As for dairy, the average serving size is eight ounces, such as an eight-ounce cup of milk.

When you add anything to your meals, get into the practice of reading the labels. My rule of thumb is to limit yourself to one serving, as identified on the label. Junk food especially—it's okay to spoil yourself once in a while, just as long as you don't go overboard.

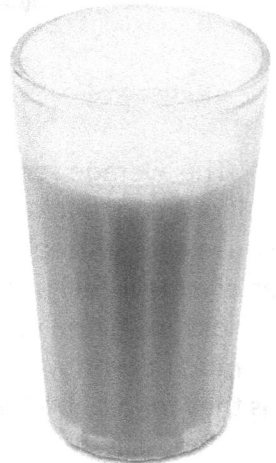

LEARN HOW TO READ NUTRITION LABELS.

Have you heard of macronutrients? Perhaps not by that technical name—you may know them as carbohydrates, proteins, and fats. Basically, macronutrients are the compounds from food that are used and stored as energy.

Carbohydrates (carbs): Every carb gram is equivalent to four calories.

Protein: Every gram of protein is equivalent to four calories.

Fats: Every gram of fat is equivalent to nine calories.

Nutrition Facts	
Serving Size ##g	
Amount Per Serving	
Calories 182	Calories from Fat 18
	% Daily Value*
Carbohydrate 35g	
Dietary Fiber 10g	
Sugars 6g	
Protein 6g	
Sodium 7mg	
Total Fat 2g	
Saturated Fat 0g	
Monounsaturated fat 1g	

*Percent Daily Values are based on a 2,000 calorie diet. Your daily values may be higher or lower depending on your calorie needs.

These are the only three things that contribute to the total calorie count of a food. So if you take the calories listed on a nutritional label from the carb, protein, and fat categories and add them up, they should equal the total calories at the top of the label. They may be off slightly due to rounding, but they should be close.

The total number of calories in this item is 182. You get this number by adding:

(fat x 9) + (carbohydrates x 4) + (protein x 4) = calories

You can do that by completing this equation:

(fat grams (F) x 9) + (carbohydrates (C) x 4) + (proteins (P) x 4) = 182

(2 g of F x 9 = 18) + (35 g of C x 4 = 140) + (6 g of P x 4 = 24)

18 + 140 + 24 = 182

Nutrition Facts

Serving Size   ##g

Amount Per Serving

Calories 182   Calories from Fat 18

% Daily Value*

Carbohydrate 35g

Dietary Fiber 10g

Sugars   6g

Protein 6g

Sodium 7mg

Total Fat   2g

Saturated Fat 0g

Monounsaturated fat 1g

*Percent Daily Values are based on a 2,000 calorie diet. Your daily values may be higher or lower depending on your calorie needs.

PAY ATTENTION
TO MEAL TIMING.

You should try to eat your meals on a set schedule. That's not always possible, thanks to life, but try to do your best—as long as you get your caloric intake for the day without going too long between eating (and slipping into starvation mode), you should be okay. Just don't double up on meals—overeating at one meal does not pay dividends, so if you have to, chalk one up as lost, and eat the next meal as planned.

Your most important meal of the day is right when you wake up. Then eat every two to four hours, depending on what you've figured out is best for your body's processing abilities through keeping your journal.

Err on the side of having most of your day's grains and breads earlier in the morning, to fuel energy levels through the day and immediately after exercising. Also, eat your largest meal of the day one to two hours before exercising.

As for your last meal of the day, it should be at least two to three hours prior to bed. This meal should contain the least amount of breads and grains, which you don't want to be stored as extra calories overnight.

AVOID THESE "SUCCESS KILLERS."

Here's the bad news: usually, the better something tastes, the worse it is for your health. When you're hooked on high-fat and high-sugar items, plain healthy food can taste bland in comparison.

This is because your body has become addicted to food sensations—the "high" of the taste, much like an addict gets an irresistible sensation from drugs. I know this is a very dramatic comparison, but it is a very real one.

Just know that as you begin switching to less-processed foods, you will experience this loss of flavor. But trust me on this—once your body recovers from the processed-food addiction, healthy "cleaner" foods will begin to taste amazing. You will crave them, in fact.

Speaking of cravings, as you wean yourself off the junk, you will experience them. For the sake of your goals, you need to fight them. When you feel a craving, try drinking a large amount of water. Or eat vegetables. It won't taste the same, obviously, but it can help trigger a "full" response in

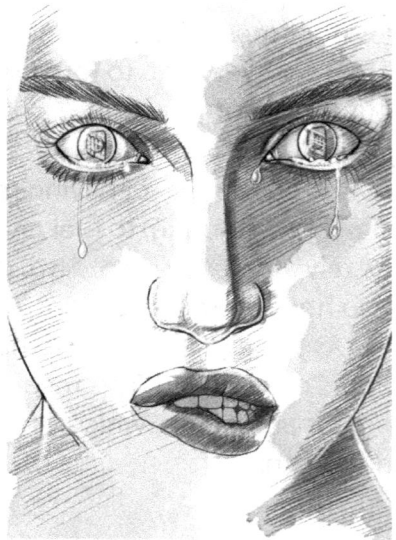

your stomach that can help you get past it. Every overcome craving is a small victory leading up to the larger one.

The main things to avoid are processed foods, like what you find at fast-food joints. If you want to see what I mean, go in and ask for a nutritional menu. You'll see some extremely high calorie counts. That's because the foods have been prepared to maximize the "addictive" flavor, using sugars and fats.

Sugar, it seems, is everywhere: drinks, candy, pastries, and places you wouldn't necessarily expect. It goes back to reading nutritional labels.

This brings us to a common question: Doesn't fruit also have sugar in it? Yes, it does, but it is a different type than the typical sugar found in processed foods. That's table sugar, or sucrose. Fruit sugar is fructose, a natural sugar that isn't as fattening and harmful as table sugar. The body more easily digests it.

Note that "bad" sugars are usually mixed into the so-called "all-natural fruit drinks." Read the label and see what percentage of real juice is actually in that bottle. Chances are, it's not much, whereas there is plenty of table sugar in the mix.

This packet of sugar is equivalent roughly to two grams of sugar. Consider this every time you go to eat or drink something containing high levels of sugar.

The single serving of soda is twelve ounces. A twelve-ounce glass of soda contains an average of thirty-nine grams of sugar in a sin-gle serving. The cup next to it also contains thirty-nine grams of sugar, in the original sugar form. Just think of that next

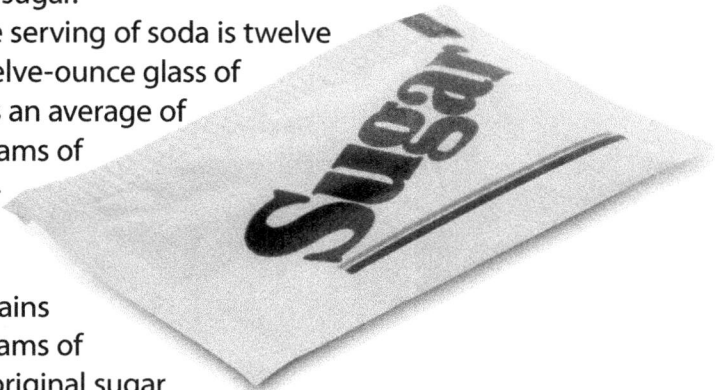

time you drink a cola—that's what you're putting in your body! Then put it down, as quickly as you can, and switch to good old water.

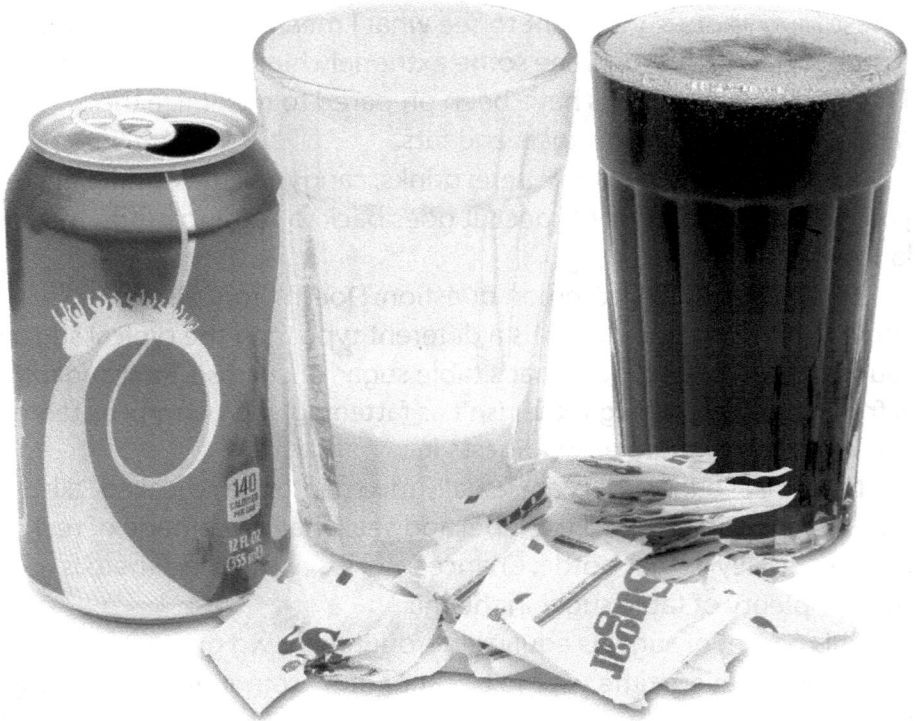

STRETCH YOURSELF.

Stretching can be a very beneficial activity, but that doesn't mean most people do it. In fact, even plenty of athletes tend to skip it or at least give it short shrift in their training.

In my view, everyone should stretch three times a day at a minimum: when you wake up, before you exercise, and after you exercise. Each stretching session should last at least five to ten minutes. If you're not familiar with specific stretching techniques, you can research them on the Internet or in the fitness section of your local library or bookstore.

Stretching is important because it increases flexibility and lowers the risk of suffering an injury. Stretching also increases the blood flow to the muscles, which allows for faster removal of lactic acid (a by-product of exercise) and delivery of nutrients from the blood to muscles, speeding up the recovery process. Stretching also warms up the muscles, making them limber and ready for action.

FIND WHAT YOU LIKE
AND GET ACTIVE.

Now that you've begun to eat healthier and started stretching, it's time for you to figure out your preferred mode of exercise. Ask yourself what activities you most   enjoy.

The exercise you choose needs to be fun for you, something that allows you to mentally relax. Exercise should be enjoyable, a place and time for you to release the stress and frustration you have built up. Exercise can be anything from a slow walk to an intense game of pickup basketball. As long as you are actively doing something that gets your heart rate up and

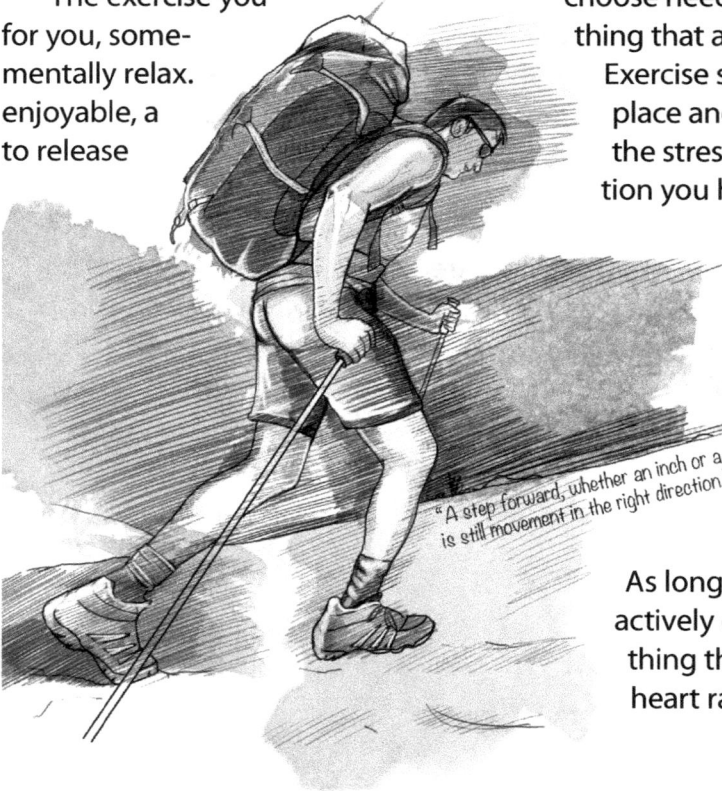

"A step forward, whether an inch or a leap is still movement in the right direction."

your body moving vigorously, you are progressively moving forward. A step forward, whether it's an inch or a mile, is still a step forward in the right direction.

If you don't know what you enjoy, go try an exercise or a sport. If you find you're not a fan of it, go try a different one. Try them all and then decide what you would like to do. This is why almost all gyms and sports clubs have a free trial period. Plus, even trying the sport or exercise is still exercise, so you're still moving forward.

When you finally decide what you like, schedule time to do it regularly. You want to exercise anywhere from twenty to sixty minutes per session, four or five times per week. You can do more than that if you like, but try to do at least the minimum of twenty minutes a day, four days a week. These minimums are at least enough to induce some muscle growth and calorie burning.

If you are eating properly and exercising four times a week, you should begin to see your body start to make positive changes. You'll feel healthier, have more energy, and be less mentally stressed. At first, your muscles may ache after exercise, but as you build up tolerance, your body adjusts, and these pains fade. Eventually, you will strive for those aches, as an indication that you've had a great workout!

EASE YOUR WAY
INTO ACTIVITY.

If exercising is new to you, the best way to get started is to ease your way into it. Set small short-term goals—just enough to ensure that every time you go out to exercise, you're going just a bit farther then you did last time. One more rep or a little more weight if you're weight training, or five more minutes or a little more distance if you're doing something cardiovascular in nature. This is where the drive to become a better person needs to kick in. All it takes is just that tiny push.

For example, say your goal revolves around doing push-ups each day. On the first day, you manage two push-ups. That's okay…as they say, it's a start! Don't get discouraged.

Next time, do your best to get three repetitions. Once you get three, try for four in the next session, and so on. This way, every time you exercise, you are constantly striving to increase your physical ability. An inch or a mile, it's still progress.

Just think about it: if you only add one push-up a week to your total count, by the end of the year, that's at least fifty-four push-ups. Now, can you imagine two or three years down the road? You will be a different person!

Improving your fitness and health is a marathon, not a sprint, so don't expect instant results. Pace yourself. You may actually feel weaker before you get stronger—as long as you stay in the race, you'll always be bettering yourself. Even if you take three steps forward and two steps back, you still made it one step forward, which is closer than before.

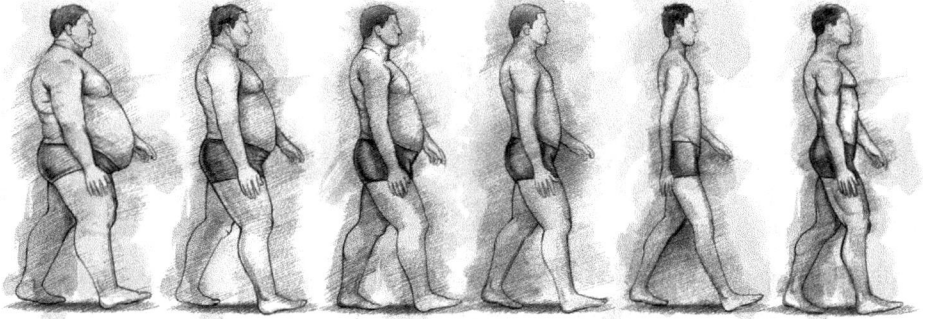

GET YOUR ZZZZ'S
AT NIGHT

For most of us in today's hectic times, the idea of resting sounds like it'll take up too much time...time you could be using to get stuff done.

But most of us underestimate the importance of sleep. The human body does all its recovery during the sleeping hours. And under times of great stress or physical strain, your body actually requires more sleep. Rest is what gives us that recharge, allowing us to stay at the top of our games. A good rest and recovery raises our level of spirits, alertness, and overall health.

Think of those days when you wake up, and it's so hard to get out of bed. You feel sluggish, weak, slow, or agitated, and you don't want to deal with anything or anyone. You even get upset when your feet get tangled in your blankets while you're trying to swing out and plant them on the floor.

Contrast that to the days when you get a good night's sleep. The ones where you wake up with a can-do attitude, and out of nowhere you decide to rip your house apart and clean everything. Or you decide to get up and go do something, because for some reason you just feel like you woke up on the right side of the bed.

If you don't allow your body to recover, you won't allow your muscles to grow. Your body needs sleep to properly dispose of that fat you need to shed or fight off that cold that's going around. Have you ever noticed that you always feel the skinniest or healthiest first thing in the morning after a good night's sleep?

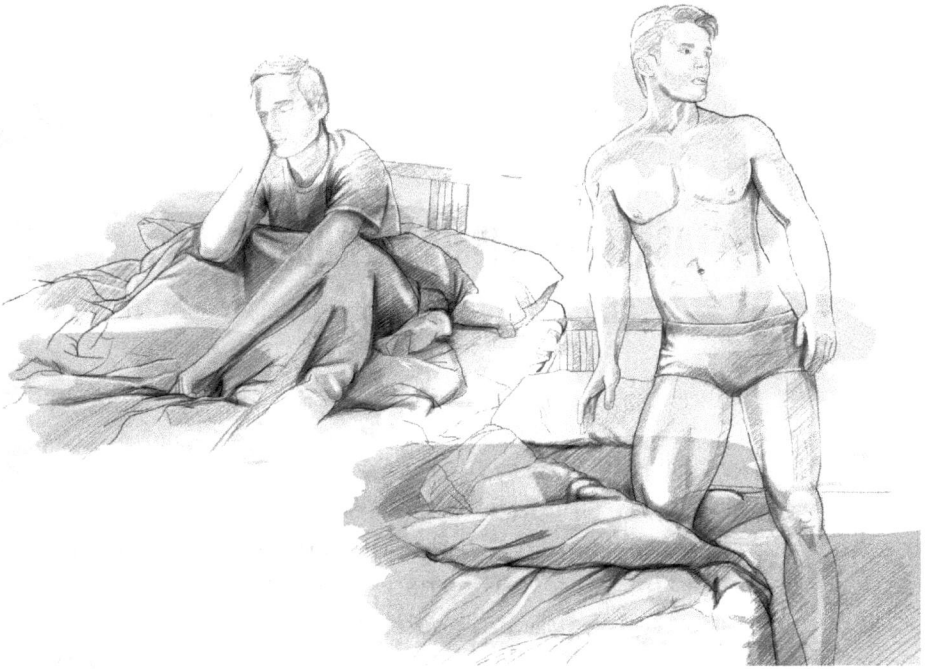

On average, your body requires eight hours of sleep a night. During stressful periods, your body requires up to nine hours of sleep. Consider this full eight- or nine-hour sleep cycle as a gas gauge, one that measures "full" as 100 percent performance.

So if you sleep only three-fourths of that, then you will only be performing at 75 percent. Such a situation is no good when your workday and workouts require 110 percent of your abilities.

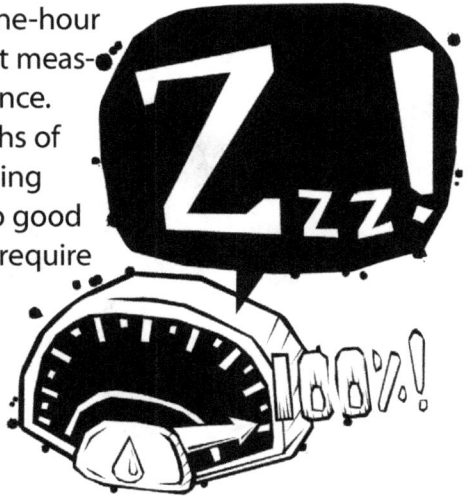

EMBRACE YOUR INNER PRESCHOOLER, AND NAP DURING THE DAY.

Napping? I know what you're saying: "I wish!"

We don't do it in the United States, but some of the other countries make time for it—a time right after lunch when all the shops close so that everyone can rest. They're onto something.

If you're tired and sluggish and need a good pick-me-up, take a nap instead of taking another hit of caffeine. Keep it to twenty or thirty minutes, and it'll give you a nice recharge. If you sleep longer than thirty minutes, however, you will fall into a deeper sleep that will be much harder to recover from.

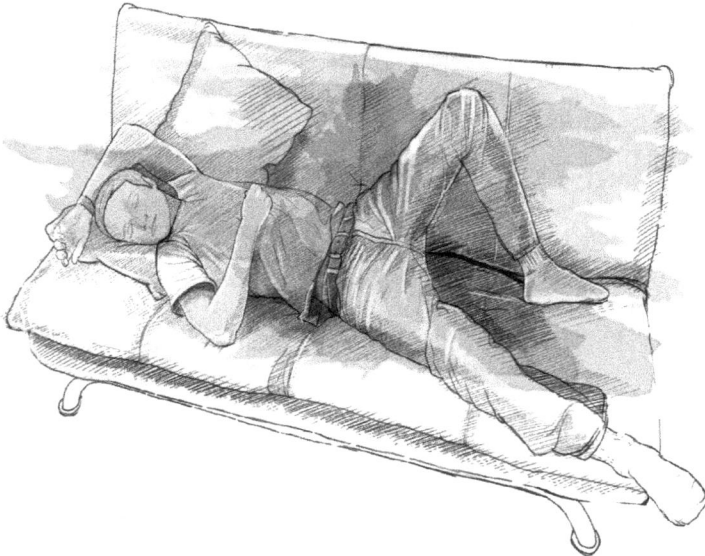

IN CONCLUSION: EIGHT KEY NOTES

Looking for a "quick list" of lifestyle changes to make? In my view, these are the key takeaways of this book:

1. Drink one ounce of water for every two pounds you weigh.

2. Sleep eight to nine hours a day. If you get a chance to nap, do so no longer than thirty minutes.

3. Eat five to seven times a day, and know what you're putting into your body is good, clean, and healthy.

4. Eat proper portions, and avoid seconds. Overeating creates fat people!

5. Whenever possible, avoid processed foods and foods containing high levels of sugar.

6. Don't eat two to three hours prior to bedtime.

7. Stretch when you wake up, begin to exercise, and when you finish an exercise routine.

8. Smile…it spreads happiness.

ABOUT THE AUTHOR

Jonathan Paul Ankiewicz was born on a military base in Germany while his father was in the Army. At the age of two he returned to the States, and he was raised in New Hampshire. He joined the US Marine Corps right out of high school. During his stint in the Marines, he was deployed to Iraq. He was also in charge of the weight-loss group for two units. After the military, he became an executive security specialist and continues to be a fitness enthusiast. He holds a Fitness Training and Specialist in Fitness Nutrition certification and is a nationally registered EMT.

www.ingramcontent.com/pod-product-compliance
Lightning Source LLC
Chambersburg PA
CBHW060528280326
41933CB00014B/3115